T0193234

A PATH TO A FIT AND HEALTHY LIFE

FOR BEGINNERS

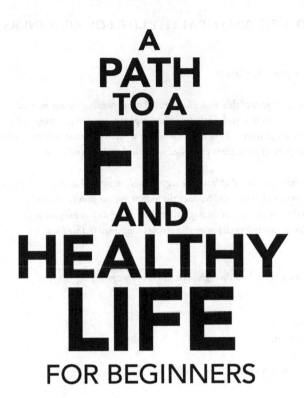

JAMES L. BLAKE JR.

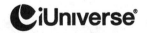

A PATH TO A FIT AND HEALTHY LIFE FOR BEGINNERS

iUniverse books may be ordered through booksellers or by contacting:

iUniverse
1663 Liberty Drive
Bloomington, IN 47403
www.iuniverse.com
1-800-Authors (1-800-288-4677)

ISBN: 978-1-5320-8402-7 (sc)
ISBN: 978-1-5320-8403-4 (e)

Library of Congress Control Number: 2019914661

Print information available on the last page.

iUniverse rev. date: 10/16/2019

CONTENTS

ACKNOWLEDGMENTS

Many people have influenced me, inspired me, and contributed to my success in life. I have to thank my mom, who, as a single parent of five, started out with little to nothing but made sure that we were informed, educated, disciplined, and pillars of society. My big sister (now deceased) always took care of me and at times was like a mother to me. She always steered me in the right direction when I would stray. Grandparents and great-uncles were there for me, providing wisdom and lessons that sometimes are overlooked.

I have to thank my immediate family—my wife and children—for always supporting me and being there throughout my military career, which was not easy, given that I was absent most of the time. My teachers were influential by supporting my ideas and believing in me. I had some male mentors in my life who were always positive, including coaches; they knew what mentoring meant to a young kid. As a soldier, I had strong leaders who were positive and knowledgeable, which helped me to become a strong leader and successful in the army.

As for my Soldiers and civilian coworkers, I thank you for your support and for testing my programs to see if they were effective. Finally, to those who always believed in me, I want to say that strength comes from within, but when you are surrounded by believers, the sky is not the limit. There is no limit.

PREFACE

For so many years, I have listened and heard people complain about their weight challenges and then look for instant results. There are no wonder pills we can take; the only way to get results is to believe that we can do it on our own. There are so many different types of programs and food charts that it is impossible to say which one is best for us. How do we choose? Anyone who has tried a program or a diet (or several programs and diets) probably has become frustrated and quit because of the lack of results. Some of us may choose to hire a personal trainer. As good as that might sound, the results still can be frustrating—and we are paying for it.

Concerns with your health and weight can be overwhelming, especially at certain times or when you're in a certain place or situation in your life. The journey is lonely, and the entire journey can become a routine that is not fulfilling or complete. You may experience many feelings and emotions when you're concerned about your health and weight, and perhaps the worst of them are depression and lack of self-esteem.

Others may try to make you feel good, or they might tell you that this book will make you into the person you want to be. This book, however, is not intended to make you feel good; it is for you to make yourself feel good, with a self-confidence that can conquer depression and boost self-esteem.

This book is partly a result of my more than thirty years of physical training and food experimentation. As a veteran with over thirty years in the United States Army and a former athlete, I can guarantee that your hard work will pay off in the long run. Knowledge is the key. You have the ability to develop an exercise and diet program that will allow you to provide your children with this insight when they are young.

I am fascinated with how to make your body work for you. Are you?

THE MIND

There are many steps to a healthy life. To choose a healthy life, you have to start with your mind. You are an extraordinary creation. You are gifted with a tool called the mind that can perform wonders. Humans can create a world of virtue or vice, pleasure or pain, from their own minds. When you understand the human mechanism and particularly the mind, which controls it, there is no limit to the heights you can climb. Your mind can enable you to acquire riches, better health, and, eventually, happiness. Whatever the mind of humankind can conceive and believe, it can achieve.

You can make and alter your outer conditions by your thoughts and feelings, with the unique gift you have to determine good from bad. You also could prevent destructive stimuli from getting into your system so that you can feed into the constructive forces that will carry your life in the right direction. Although you have inherited this mind power as a gift, you still may get entangled in worldly doubts and fears. Certain limitations that you force on yourself—such as saying, "I cannot change," "There is no use in trying," "I am unfit"—make the mind powerless to produce action. Relax your physical self and feed positive affirmations to your mind to break the cocoon and emerge as a beautiful butterfly. You are *mind* and body, not *body* and mind. Your thought processes are the main catalyst for creating illnesses, difficulties, and disabilities, both mentally and physically. Essentially, human suffering can be overcome just by instructing the mind not to allow illnesses and difficulties.

Let me paint a picture for you: The mind controls leptin, which is a novel protein produced by fat cells. Leptin acts on the brain to reduce food intake and increase energy expenditure. It has been discovered that the brain—in particular, the hypothalamus (the part of the brain that controls appetite and weight)—makes leptin. Most human obesity appears to involve the brain's ignoring the high levels of leptin in the blood, and this happens because the key regulator in the hypothalamus is locally derived of leptin.

The brain or the mental state of mind is very important when it comes to health and fitness. You are indeed what you see of yourself and what you decide to eat. Let's start with how you see yourself. When you look in the mirror or put on those favorite clothes, what do you really see and feel? If you don't see what you want or like, then this is where you should start. Your mind needs to believe in a certain look that you want to achieve; this will start your willingness to commit to a healthy life.

Picture what you want to look like, and burn that image into your mind. This sets the boundaries that you allow yourself to have. This is done unconsciously, without your realizing at first, but later, it will become a part of your life. A former professor of medicine at Stanford University, Dr. Bruce Lipton, said the new science of epigenetics has shown that our genes are in fact controlled and manipulated by how our minds perceive and interpret our environment. In other words the mind controls 95 percent of all our actions. While this is true, you cannot help but follow the images and ideas that are placed in your mind. You have to manipulate your mind to see what you want to look like. You identify the areas that you want to improve and develop a new image on how you will look with the improvements. Now the mental image is there and the boundaries are in place.

How can you become what you eat? This is simple because most foods have an ingredients list and the amount of each nutrient per serving. If you were to eat a hamburger on a daily basis without exercising to compensate for the calories, chances are your midsection would become like the shape of a hamburger. This may seem far-fetched, but once you learn how to master your body, it will be much clearer. I am not saying that you cannot eat a hamburger; I am saying to learn how to compensate for it, and have a hamburger as a variety, not a daily meal. Your mind controls what you eat. Once again, if you set your mind with boundaries, you will be amazed at the control you can have over something as simple as a hamburger.

There likely are other foods you should have as variety instead of daily, but I decided to use hamburgers because most of the population can relate. Just as your mind pictures how tasty a jelly doughnut may be, your set boundaries allow your mind to control the thought and impulse to eat that doughnut. This is the first and most important part of obtaining and maintaining a fit and healthy life.

The mind also allows you to have staying power, which is essential to choosing a fit and healthy life. You may have heard the phrase, "Once your mind is made up, nothing can stop you." This is the same attitude you need when you choose a fit and healthy life. This gives you the will to continue when you have days of no progress, and impatience sets in. Obtaining a fit and healthy life is a long process, but it will enable you to have full control of your fitness. You have to believe in yourself before you can develop your program.

I would like to share something that seems obvious but is missed every year. The months of January to March are often dedicated to well-intended New Year's resolutions. But then the gym is packed, and you cannot get to the machine to continue your workout. What you are about to read is so simple, but most of us don't think of it when we are in the moment. This applies to both those who give up on their resolutions after three months and the dedicated workers.

The mind controls your decision to make a New Year's resolution, but most important, it controls the outcome of what you started. After the third month, when your results are minimal or your weight has increased, this is when the March syndrome kicks in. It depends on the many factors that are involved when you plan to work out and lose weight or tone up.

When you weigh more than what is required for your body frame, you will aggressively loose the weight rapidly. If your body has reached a plateau, and you cannot seem to lose any more weight, that is when the mind is the biggest factor in your workout. Your mind tells you to quit, that it's a waste of time. It asks why you are doing this and says that you are good the way you are. The one to stay away from is, "I like the way I look." If you like the way you look, you would not have made a New Year's resolution to work out and lose weight.

Control is the key, and it is control of your mind that can get you past any month. It is not easy to deceive your mind, but on the same note, it is easy for your mind to give up. When you think about something that you like, nothing can change your mind from thinking the way you do. This is the same kind of thinking you need to use when working out. You should not become discouraged when you stop losing weight. That is when you are starting to dig into who you are trying to become. Continue to focus your mind, and I promise you that by the end of your journey into the fitness world, you will not be disappointed. Your mind can transform your body in so many ways, some of which are unbelievable.

Before you start your program, it is very important to find that strong influence that keeps you on course. If you are derailed for any reason, just start at the beginning to validate what your initial goal was and the reason you committed to your program. Remember that this program is one that *you* developed, and you should be able to sustain it. Your thoughts are more important than you can imagine. You can be *fit for life.*

THE INNER BODY

The inner body is essential to a workout program. This is the core of what you are trying to become. Inner beauty is what you are trying to bring out. I believe that when your inside is feeling well, then your outside will look and feel well. The more you work on your inner body, the more successful you will be with your outer body. It is not just what you eat but also what you do not eat. It is not only what you take but also what you do not take. The types of foods that you eat are very important to your inner body. Part of developing your program is knowing which types of foods fuel your body the way that you would like. This process takes time, but the results will be rewarding.

Everybody reacts to different types of foods differently. Finding the types of foods that fuel your body in the right way is almost like finding yourself again. Take the time needed to experiment, and find the right foods for you. I also mentioned it is what you take and do not take. You may take supplements, vitamins, or weight-loss supplements to enhance or even to quicken the process or goal that you want. You may have various excuses for taking weight-loss supplements, such as,

- I didn't have time to eat properly.
- I need something to keep my energy up.
- I need help to lose weight faster.

And the excuses go on. My opinion on over-the-counter drugs is that they are a poor excuse for not finding out what kind of food your body needs for fuel. Some cases may require supplements, vitamins or weight-loss supplements, but I would ask you how it got to that point.

You need to attack a core point of fitness, which is body metabolism. With the right combinations of foods, you can help raise your metabolism. Once again, this takes time, and time is all you need when seeking a healthy life.

The plan is simple: you have to power yourself into the program, and stick with it. If you are looking for a quick-fix-solution, it won't satisfy your inner body, which can be a reflection of your outer body. The satisfaction comes from knowing you found yourself and developed and discovered something that will remain with you for a lifetime.

The other part that you want to explore is the endurance factor. Building up endurance enables you to burn body fat at a higher rate. It also expands your lung capacity to allow more oxygen flow to the blood. How does this help? The blood feeds the muscles, and the oxygen feeds the blood. Muscles need fresh, oxygenated blood so they do not tire out as fast. Expanding your lung capacity allows your muscles to remain fresh longer. This is one of the steps needed for a fit and healthy life. Building endurance takes time, but what is good about taking your time is that you simultaneously expand your lung capacity, which allows your muscles to remain fresh longer. Once again, time is all you have. After all, you are talking about being healthier and achieving your goal. Once you start building your endurance, then you will see—and more important, feel—the difference in your body. Remember that the inner body is the key to your success and should not be neglected.

You can eat almost anything you like, but your program has to be on track, and your goal must be met before you venture out or deviate from your program. Your metabolism is part of your inner body that continues to burn fat, even after you have completed your workout. When you can eat almost anything you like and maintain your achieved goal, this is when you know that you have the winning combination, and you have found yourself. You have to think of your inner body just like everything else—if you fuel it, you should use it.

Do not fuel your body with a full meal if you are not planning to use that fuel. That is one of the times when your body decides where the fuel will be stored. Your body may store the fuel in the area in which you are trying to lose weight. Make sure that your fuel intake matches your fuel expenditure. You will learn to manage your fuel intake as you continue to develop your program. Take into account that it is not only *what* you eat, but it is also *when* you eat.

THE OUTER BODY

The outer body is the visual confirmation that you have chosen a fit and healthy life. Of course, this comes with exercising. Now that your mind is set, identify your areas for improvement, and imagine how the areas will look when you have reached your goal. The idea is for you to develop your own program. Being able to develop your own program not only supports your mental boundaries, but it also builds self-confidence and high self-esteem. I want you to go the gym or to work out wherever you would like with high self-esteem and lots of self-confidence. This will also help your staying power when things do not seem to be working.

It has been said that the older you get, the slower your metabolism becomes. I believe this to be true, but this is like everything else that gets old—if you take care of it with the proper maintenance, it will last a lifetime. Your body is like a machine, and it desires the same type of maintenance— and sometimes even more.

For example, let's say you buy a brand-new car (similar to a newborn baby) that has everything checked out and is ready to drive (leave the hospital). Over the years, you change the fluids and replace them with new fluids (body excretes waste, and you eat again). You change the tires (buy new shoes), clean it up (wash the body), and have tune-ups (doctor checkups).

Now your car is older, and you are similar in so many ways. The car will last a lifetime with the right program to take care of it—and so will your body. The battery jump-starts a car, just as the cardiovascular system jump-starts your body. Your body requires your target heart rate to be raised, or elevated, at least three times a week. This pushes the blood throughout the body at an accelerated pace. If you let a car idle without movement, it will eventually run hot. If you leave a car stored for a long period without movement, the fluids will break down, and the seals will dry out and rot from lack of lubrication. It is the same for the human body; you must periodically come out of the idle state. Never sit around without having any activity in your life.

During the construction of your program, there are certain things that you should consider. When you go to the gym and see other people working out with a book or chart in their hands, this is not a program; it is a workout guide. The book and chart tell the person to follow a guide without there being any personal research, and it's supposed to be successful. I want you to have a program developed for you and by you. Having a book or chart at your side while working out won't help the development of a solid program. A workout program is something that is second nature to you, which you can develop on your own. When you go to the gym or workout area, there should be no doubt in your mind what you are about to do. Once again, this goes back to your mental state and building self-confidence and high self-esteem.

The program will not work for you if you are trying to be a body builder. This program is geared toward people who are trying to achieve one of the three levels (or all three levels) below. The three levels in the program are as follows:

1. weight loss
2. fitness
3. toning

The first level in the program is losing weight. At first, it will be easy to lose weight if you have never worked out. The cardiovascular system plays an important part in level one. When you start at level one, depending on your size, you will lose weight quickly. This is no reason to be alarmed. Continue to maintain great eating habits, and your health will be fine. Rapid weight lost is due to various reasons, but two common reasons are the increase or implementation of cardiovascular activities and the combinations of foods that contribute to weight lost. Once you have lost weight, your body will plateau and stabilize at a certain weight. If this is the desired weight, then level two is not the next step. If this is not the weight that you mentally set in your mind, then the combination of levels one and two should be used.

During the process of level one, you will have begun the steps in level two, but that was not the focus. Losing weight in level one was the focus in your program. You have to know how to stay within your program. When your body plateaus, which means that your rapid weight is gone, you have to increase your cardiovascular activity to lose more weight. The fitness chart shows how you can increase and monitor your levels. Remember, the chart does not travel with you to the gym or workout place; it is merely for you to record your results of the program that is in your mind. Also, a height-and-weight chart will be provided for you to gauge activities.

The chart may seem a little extreme in some cases, but remember that it is based on weight equally distributed throughout the body. I have experimented with the height-and-weight chart ratio on others and on myself (undocumented) and found that the burning fat and calorie metabolism is much faster when the chart ratio is met. When your metabolism speeds up, then you are able to burn fat and calories quicker. This gives you a faster recovery from that hamburger. A higher metabolism is what you want to achieve during your workout program. This is one of the goals that you are working toward.

The program that you develop is geared for your lifestyle. This is why it is very important that you understand and establish your program. The minimum amount of time you should invest in your program to see a result is thirty days. There is not a maximum amount of time for your program. The continuation is based on what you want to accomplish, your desire, and your staying power. Your program is designed so that you can adjust it as needed. It is not as complicated as it may seem, nor as complicated as others might try to imply. The program consists of your trying different techniques and foods until you find what works for you, while achieving your goal.

Don't be discouraged if you do not make your target goal in the first week. It is imperative that you continue developing your program until you find which one works for you. The program, just like everything you do, will not work without discipline. Again, that is why the mental state is the first and most important part of the program. The program starts with the mind and ends with the mind. Once you have set your mind to achieve your goal with boundaries, and you develop your program, it will always be in your mind.

Level two is automatically factored in to your program, merely by the workout you will achieve in level one. Level two has many kinds of fitness, but you should focus on the natural way to fitness. Your program will consist of cardiovascular activity, various exercises, and weight training. You select the exercises from a variety of choices that can be used separately or in combinations.

The weight training is not intended to bulk up your muscles but to help tone them. The weights with which you chose to work out should always be comfortable and not to the point where you have to strain to complete a repetition. The idea is to have low repetitions and more sets to develop tone and not bulk. Once you have found a comfortable weight for working out, maintain that weight throughout your workout. When you increase the weight, you will increase your bulk. Remember that you are working toward losing weight, getting fit, and developing toned muscles.

What is the program for level three? You already have the knowledge to develop your program for level three. Your muscles are taking on shape as you work out and develop your program. Toning comes when you are comfortable with your outer body and ready to have concentrated workouts. Level three uses toning in your program, with repetition and sets at an intense level. Remember that increasing your weight will increase your bulk, and that is not the target for the development of the program.

Why is losing weight first so important? Muscle will build with fat. This means that lifting heavy weights without losing the fat will cause the fat to become hard and give the appearance of muscle. Imagine a poorly cut steak when you first start cooking it. The steak is huge, but after cooking awhile, it is reduced in size. This is because the fat is burned away, leaving more meat than fat. Another thought is how huge a hamburger is prior to cooking it and how much smaller it becomes after cooking it. That is why you should burn away the fat in your body, so you can build the lean muscles. Fat can be good on your body, but you need to burn off the excess prior to building a fit body. Fat is an important part of your body's makeup, but too much can hurt you as well.

Your fitness is measured in many ways. One sure way to tell your fitness level is how fast your body recovers after a stressful training event. How long does it take your heart rate to return to normal after a stressful training event? A fit body is easy to tone because it's all about fine-tuning. When you fine-tune your body, it is just as important to watch what you do to the inside as the outside. An easy way to tone the outer body is to know what got you to that level of fitness. You will need to adjust your cardiovascular activity by making it longer, faster, or more intense. Refer to the fitness chart for examples. By increasing your cardiovascular activity, your fat and calories will burn at a higher rate. This will help you overcome that plateau stage.

Once again, if this is the level that you desire when you plateau, then just continue with the same program that you developed. For those who are continuing or who did not reach their goals, there are many ways to implement cardiovascular activity into your program. There are seven ways that I suggest, ranging from the most effective to the least effective. Identify which one will fit into your program and implement it. The cardiovascular exercises I recommend are (1) running, (2) walking, (3) aerobics, (4) swimming, (5) bicycling, (6) elliptical machine, and (7) Stairmaster. There also are other exercises and programs available. Again, this is about you developing your own program, at no cost except your time.

Cardiovascular activity brings endurance to the table, which enhances you're staying power to work out in your program. Endurance is helpful outside of your workout program as well, especially for those with long hours or early mornings on the job.

Running is number one because it allows total body motion. Depending on your running regimen, you can employ the majority of your large muscle groups, which take longer to develop, and your endurance will increase significantly.

Do not enter into running lightly. There is a technique to running, and it is different for each individual. Running outdoors is the preferred method, but you can run indoors as well. This offers versatility when the weather is not cooperating with you. I will address running indoors and other techniques that can be used in chapter 7. Just make sure you select the cardiovascular exercise that will fit into your program.

IMPORTANCE AND STATISTICS

You name it, and it is possible—stroke, arthritis, birth defects, breast cancer, high cholesterol, cardiovascular disease, type 2 diabetes, gall bladder disease, high blood pressure, gout, heart disorders, infertility, liver disease, and obesity. If you have one of the above-mentioned diseases, make a choice in life.

Once you have chosen a healthy life, consult your doctor before you start any training program. You can prevent weight gain by assessing your behavior and environment. The amount and type of foods you eat and your physical activity are important factors in controlling weight. The environment in which you live may contribute to poor eating and exercise habits. The US Surgeon General recommends moderate physical activity on most days of the week, at least thirty minutes per day for adults and sixty minutes per day for children.

Because the mind plays a major role in avoiding obesity and in choosing a healthy life, it's important to understand the facts about obesity. Obesity is a complex, multifactorial chronic disease involving environmental (social and cultural), genetic, physiologic, metabolic, behavioral, and psychological components. It is a chronic condition that is more simply defined as an excess amount of body fat. It is the second cause of preventable death in the United States, coming in a close second to tobacco.

Obesity is a complex health issue that results from a combination of causes and contributing factors, including behavior and genetics. Behavior can include dietary patterns, physical activity, inactivity, medication use, and other exposures. Additional contributing factors in society include the food and physical-activity environment, education and skills, and food marketing and promotion (CDC 2017).

Obesity is a serious concern because it is associated with poorer mental health outcomes and reduced quality of life. It is one of the leading causes of death in the United States and worldwide, including diabetes, heart disease, stroke, and some types of cancer (CDC 2017).

PHILOSOPHICAL VIEW

I cannot begin to express the importance of being healthy throughout your life on this earth. You may take it for granted most of the time, until something of great significance happens in your life. Usually, it is a *significant emotional event* (SEE), death of a close loved one, or near death for you.

I consider not being healthy and not maintaining fitness in your life as self-inflicted stress. Self-inflicted stress is something that you can control about yourself and that can be prevented. If high blood pressure runs in your family that does not mean that you will automatically have high blood pressure. You already have the advantage by knowing your family's medical history. That is why it is self-inflicted stress when you allow the same illness to happen to you. You can set boundaries and control your existence here on earth. You are able to attack and accomplish the things you want in life; you should take the same attitude toward your health and fitness. You may get caught up in the society that is life-driven. By the time you realize what is going on in your life, it is too late. Wake up to the reality, not before it is too late for you but before it is too late for your children.

Think of the lives of your ancestors. They likely ate whatever foods they wanted each day. How was it possible for them and their children to survive without the diabetes, high blood pressure, heart disease, and all the health problems that many of us deal with today? It's because most of the jobs back then were manual labor that required daily physicality. This is not the makeup of most jobs today.

You are giving a free will to pursue the type of life you choose. One myth is that healthy equates to wealthy. This is only part of the equation: healthy + wealthy = happiness. If you take this equation and apply it to society, then the results will be what they are now. You may try to fix this mode of thinking because your kids are the victims of this equation.

First, the word *healthy* needs to be defined; what is it, and what is being healthy? Then look at the word *wealthy*, which will have different meanings for different people. Wealthy is dependent upon healthy if you plan on enjoying any of that wealth. Then there's *happiness*, which is the one thing that everyone desires. Happiness is spun off both healthy and wealthy; being happy simply means living a healthy life and having enough wealth to provide for yourself and your family.

The equation is very simple; you have to be the active party when it comes to your fitness. All the money in the world cannot bring you fitness or happiness unless you are active in what makes your body prone to a fit and healthy life.

Reflect on your life, thoroughly considering your happiest times and your saddest times. What was your status and how was your health? Take the time to consider your past to help push you in the direction that you want to go.

There are secrets that are not mentioned in most training, but they are something you do every day. Think about when you get up from a chair; you use your legs or arms. What about when you are sitting for a long time? Do you try to hold your stomach in for sixty seconds at least every thirty seconds? One of the big secrets to being fit and healthy is continuous exercise that is seamless with what you are doing.

Here is how it is done: compare your exercise in your program to your everyday lifestyle, and make the everyday lifestyle a part of your routine. The triceps muscle is used when you lift yourself out of the chair—that could be a part of your continuous exercise program. This is only one example. The challenge is for you to continue to develop your program. This can be the beginning of a new life adventure for you.

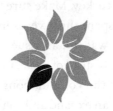

THE FOOD CHART

This is the part of your program that is often overlooked or ignored. Developing your program includes a food program. You cannot have control of your body unless you commit to the food program, which you will develop on your own. You will start with a baseline of food groups, but you will have to experiment with the combinations to find your appropriate diet. Again, this is a thirty-day process. The following chart is an example of how to set up your weekly food groups and combinations. (You have to decide which combinations work for your body.)

Days	Week One	Week Two	Week Three	Week Four
Meals	Breakfast: oat/bran cereal or bagel	Breakfast: oat/bran cereal or bagel	Breakfast: oat/bran cereal or bagel	Breakfast: oat/bran cereal or bagel
Substitute salad for tuna	Lunch: tuna & crackers; fruit for snacks	Lunch: tuna & crackers; fruit for snacks	Lunch: tuna & crackers; fruit for snacks	Lunch: tuna & crackers; fruit for snacks
No fried foods	Dinner: baked chicken with noodles & veg	Dinner: baked fish with veg only	Dinner: baked chicken with noodles & veg	Dinner: baked fish with veg only
Drink a lot of water	Breakfast: a glass of juice is allowed	Lunch: turkey subs are good with oil/vinegar	Dinner should be eaten by 8:00 p.m., or salad only	Smoothies are good also

What other foods can you add to your group? For the meal rotations, you can also try salmon and turkey. Make sure to expand the vegetable and fruit range to your liking. I spent three years in Italy. The people there ate pasta every day, and weight was not an issue. This was their culture; you would have to develop yours. Instead of pasta, rice may be your thing. Again, it is up to you to figure out the combinations that fit you. Remember to achieve your goal; then you can expand and splurge a little. Can you control portion sizes of your food intake? Yes, look at your portion size before you start eating. The formula is simple: if you have two spoonful of rice, reduce it to one and one half spoonful of rice. Reduce two pieces of chicken to one and a half pieces of chicken. Continue to do this, once you find out your working food group. The objective is to find the food group that works; then starts reducing your portions slowly. It is important that you do not rush the reducing process. Developing a program takes time. (Wait until you plateau out.)

EXERCISE CHART

The exercise charts are designed for each individual. These charts will help you develop your own workout program that you can manage. Many fitness programs today are mainly for the persons who developed them. No one person is the same as someone else; therefore, no one person can develop a complete fitness program for another person without doing thorough research—and that takes time. If you want to pay personal trainer money for something that you can develop and understand by yourself, it is your choice. Your responsibility should be to know about your body and learn what makes your body responds. The program that you develop will help you figure it out.

I will explain how to develop your own workout program that supports not only your body but your work schedule. Time is never a factor if you read chapter 1 and realize that positive thinking will allow you to find the appropriate time for you. Morning would be my first choice, to allow the body to burn calories all day and have time to recover if you choose a daily workout. My second choice would be lunchtime because that still allows your body the time to continue to burn calories and recover. Dinnertime would be my last choice; your state of mind after a long day of working may not be ideal. A workout, regardless of the time, will always do more good than harm, if you know what you are doing.

You may think that it is not possible for you to manage your own fitness chart and develop a program. This chart, along with the program you develop from this chart, will show you results within thirty days. Your program cannot be aggressive if you are a beginner. The charts are based on the average person but can be lowered, if needed, to have a less aggressive start. Allow yourself time to plan your workout before starting. This will prevent you from having minor injuries that will stop your workout after you get into it.

Let me help you put away the books and papers you may have carried to the gym. Your mind is where the program needs to be—embedded. It is very simple; you figure out your target, and attack it with the goal to conquer. Look at the outcome, not the beginning. The outcome must be in your mind for you to be successful.

Take the midsection, for example. More and more people wear low-cut jeans and tight shirts with their stomachs hanging out. That is not the look you should try to achieve with this program. The program is for you to achieve the fit look. You can design your program to be more abdominal-intensive, if that is what you desire. This is why this program will work for each individual and not stereotype everyone.

The chart is simple to use. You input your fitness status and make improvements at your own pace. For example, if you are doing ten push-ups in the first week, then your number of push-ups should increase from ten to fifteen in the second week. This method applies to every exercise that you do while developing your program.

Another example: if your walk time is thirty minutes for two miles in the first week, then your walk time for the following week should be less than thirty minutes. This same method is applied to running and other exercises suggested on the charts. If you keep applying this technique to your workout until you reach your goal, you will develop your program while achieving your goal. Running or walking inside on a track is similar to doing it outside but the adjustments are the rotations around the track to achieve the same goals. Using the treadmill inside is not difficult for running or walking it takes some knowledge of the equipment. Knowing your pace for running or walking will allow you to program the machine to your desired pace and miles. The treadmill is the closest thing to running outside and is needed sometimes when the weather does not permit outside activities.

The program that you are developing is for you and only you. Remember: everyone is different. It's up to you to find out what works for you. The chart is provided for you to make adjustments and changes to fit your workout needs.

A PATH TO A FIT AND HEALTHY LIFE FOR BEGINNERS

The exercise chart and food chart are suggestions and examples of how to start your path to a fit life for beginners.

Walkers

Days	Week One	Week Two	Week Three	Week Four
Monday	2M/36MIN 25 P/U & 25 S/U	2M/34MIN ___ P/U & ___ S/U	2M/30MIN ___ P/U & ___ S/U	2M/28MIN 50 P/U & 50 S/U
Tuesday	BIKE AT LEVEL 10, 80 RPM FOR 10M, 100 CRUNCHES, 100 SUPINE BICYCLE	BIKE AT LEVEL 10, 80 RPM FOR 10M, 100 CRUNCHES, 100 SUPINE BICYCLE	BIKE AT LEVEL 10, 80 RPM FOR 10M, 100 CRUNCHES, 100 SUPINE BICYCLE	BIKE AT LEVEL 10, 80 RPM FOR 10M, 100 CRUNCHES, 100 SUPINE BICYCLE
Wednesday	2M/36MIN 25 P/U & 25 S/U	2M/34MIN ___ P/U & ___ S/U	2M/30MIN ___ P/U & ___ S/U	2M/28MIN 50 P/U & 50 S/U
Thursday	BIKE AT LEVEL 10, 80 RPM FOR 10M, 100 CRUNCHES, 100 SUPINE BICYCLE	BIKE AT LEVEL 10, 80 RPM FOR 10M, 100 CRUNCHES, 100 SUPINE BICYCLE	BIKE AT LEVEL 10, 80RPM FOR 10M, 100 CRUNCHES, 100 SUPINE BICYCLE	BIKE AT LEVEL 10, 80RPM FOR 10M, 100 CRUNCHES, 100 SUPINE BICYCLE
Friday	2M/36MIN 25 P/U & 25 S/U	2M/34MIN ___ P/U & ___ S/U	2M/30MIN ___ P/U & ___ S/U	2M/28MIN 50 P/U & 50 S/U
Saturday (Optional)	2M/36MIN 25 P/U & 25 S/U	2M/34MIN ___ P/U & ___ S/U	2M/30MIN ___ P/U & ___ S/U	2M/28MIN ___ P/U & ___ S/U
Sunday	REST	REST	REST	REST
Meals	B/F: oat/bran cereal or bagel	B/F: oat/bran cereal or bagel	B/F: oat/bran cereal or bagel	B/F: oat/bran cereal or bagel
Substitute salad for tuna	L: tuna & crackers; fruits for snacks	L: tuna & crackers; fruits for snacks	L: tuna & crackers; fruits for snacks	L: tuna & crackers; fruits for snacks
No fried foods	D: baked chicken with noodles & veg	D: baked fish with veg only	D: baked chicken with noodles & veg	D: baked fish with veg only
Drink a lot of water	B/F: a glass of juice is allowed	L: turkey subs are good with oil/vinegar	D: meals eaten by 8:00 p.m., or salad only	Smoothies are good also

P/U = push-ups; S/U = sit-ups; M = miles; MIN = minutes; B/F = breakfast; L = lunch; D = dinner

Note: The time is flexible and based on the initial time on Monday. You should try to increase your P/U and S/U time every week. If your time Monday is 28MIN, then the week-two goal should be 26MIN. Always try to decrease or maintain. These are just the minimums that must be kept; any additional exercise is welcomed. Continue to decrease the time and increase the distance. *It's important to stretch before and after exercises.*

Runners

Days	Week One	Week Two	Week Three	Week Four
Monday	2M/__MIN 25 P/U & 25 S/U	3M/30MIN ___ P/U & ___ S/U	3M/27MIN ___ P/U & ___ S/U	4M/36MIN 50 P/U & 50 S/U
Tuesday	BIKE AT LEVEL10, 80RPM FOR 10M, 100 CRUNCHES, 100 SUPINE BICYCLE	BIKE AT LEVEL10, 80RPM FOR 10M, 100 CRUNCHES, 100 SUPINE BICYCLE	BIKE AT LEVEL10, 80RPM FOR 10M, 100 CRUNCHES, 100 SUPINE BICYCLE	BIKE AT LEVEL10, 80RPM FOR 10M, 100 CRUNCHES, 100 SUPINE BICYCLE
Wednesday	2M/-30 SEC 25 P/U & 25 S/U	3M/-30 SEC ___ P/U & ___ S/U	3M/-30 SEC ___ P/U & ___ S/U	4M/-30 SEC 50 P/U & 50 S/U
Thursday	BIKE AT LEVEL10, 80RPM FOR 10M, 100 CRUNCHES, 100 SUPINE BICYCLE	BIKE AT LEVEL10, 80RPM FOR 10M, 100 CRUNCHES, 100 SUPINE BICYCLE	BIKE AT LEVEL10, 80RPM FOR 10M, 100 CRUNCHES, 100 SUPINE BICYCLE	BIKE AT LEVEL10, 80RPM FOR 10M, 100 CRUNCHES, 100 SUPINE BICYCLE
Friday	2M/-30 SEC 25 P/U & 25 S/U	3M/-30 SEC ___ P/U & ___ S/U	3M/-30 SEC ___ P/U & ___ S/U	4M/-30 SEC 50 P/U & 50 S/U
Saturday (Optional)	2M/___MIN 25 P/U & 25 S/U	3M/___MIN ___ P/U & ___ S/U	3M/___MIN ___ P/U & ___ S/U	4M/___MIN ___ P/U & ___ S/U
Sunday	REST	REST	REST	REST
Meals	B/F: oat/bran cereal or bagel	B/F: oat/bran cereal or bagel	B/F: oat/bran cereal or bagel	B/F: oat/bran cereal or bagel
Substitute salad for tuna	L: tuna & crackers; fruits for snacks	L: tuna & crackers; fruits for snacks	L: tuna & crackers; fruits for snacks	L: tuna & crackers; fruits for snacks
No fried foods	D: baked chicken with noodles & veg	D: baked fish with veg only	D: baked chicken with noodles & veg	D: baked fish with veg only
Drink a lot of water	B/F: a glass of juice is allowed	L: turkey subs are good with oil/vinegar	D: meals eaten by 8:00 p.m., or salad only	

P/U=PUSH UPS; S/U=SIT UPS; M=MILES; MIN=MINUTES; B/F=BREAKFAST; L=LUNCH; D=DINNER;

Note: This time is flexible and based on the initial time on Monday. You should try to increase your P/U and S/U every week. Always try to increase or maintain. These are just the minimums that must be kept; any additional exercise is welcomed. Continue to decrease the time and increase the distance. *It's important to stretch before and after exercises.*

The following are additional exercises that can help with the development of your individual plan. I did not supply you with exercise pictures, because it is a valuable part of your research.

	Monday	Tuesday	Wednesday	Thursday	Friday	Saturday
Side Straddle Hop 25/4 count.........						
Cross Country Skier 25/4 count.........						
Ski Jumper 25/4 count.........						
Abdominal Crunch (Legs at 90 Degrees Hands Behind Head Holding Base of the Neck and Back/Feet Flat. Lift Upper Shoulders to Crunch Abdominal.) 25 count........						
Regular Crunch with Legs Up 25 count.......						
Supine Bicycle 15/4 count.....						
Flutter Kicks 15/4 count.....						
Leg Spreader Crossover 15/4 count.......						
Regular Push Ups 25 count........						
Front/Right/Left Pilates 25 sec count........						
Knee to Elbow (Standing with your Hands Behind your Head Fingers Interlock, Legs Shoulder with apart, Bring your Right Elbow to your Left Knee then your Left Elbow to your Right Knee but not touching) 25/4 count each.......						
Reverse Dips 10-25 count....................						
Chin Up Hold 25 sec count (optional)......						
Pull Ups 10 count (optional)...........						
Hanging Crunches 10 count (optional)...........						
The Key is to complete Three (3) sets in this order with only 60 seconds or less between the three sets.						

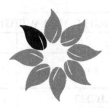

CHART (BURNING METABOLISM)

Provided is an example of a male and female, 20 pounds (lbs.) over the burning metabolism (BM) height (HT) and weight (WT) scale. If you gain 20 pounds over the BM for each age group, your weight can still be managed by maintaining body fat (BF) percentage of 20% or less for males, and 25% or less for females. The BF percentage should descend by 2% for each age group for the max allowed, with 20% and 25% being the max. The blank spaces on the following chart were left intentionally.

Height and Weight Chart (burning metabolism)

BURNING METABOLISM/HEIGHT AND WEIGHT FOR MALE AND FEMALE							
HEIGHT (in inches)	Male Age				Example Max WT with BF%		
	17 - 20	21 - 28	28 - 39	40+			
	BURNING WEIGHT				WT + Pds =	Total WT	<=20%
54	95 - 100	100 - 105	105 - 110	110 - **115**			
55	100 - 105	105 - 110	110 - 115	115 - 120			
56	100 - 105	105 - 110	110 - 115	115 - 120			
57	105 - 110	110 - 115	115 - 12 0	120 - 125			
58	110 - 115	115 - 120	120 - 125	125 - 130			
59	115- 120	120 - 125	125 - 130	130 - 135			
6 0	120 - 125	125 - 130	130 - 135	135 - 140			
6 1	125 - 130	130 - 135	135 - 140	140 - 145			
6 2	130 - 135	135 - 140	140 - 145	145 - 150			
6 3	135- 140	140 - 145	145 - 150	150 - 155			
6 4	140 - 145	145 - 150	150 - 155	155 - 160			
6 5	145- 150	150 - 155	155 - 160	160 - 165			
6 6	150 -155	155 - 160	160 - 165	165 - 170			
6 7	155 - 160	160 - 165	165 - 170	170 - 175			
6 8	160 - 165	165 - 170	170 -175	175 - 180			
6 9	160 - 165	165 - 170	170 - 175	175 - 185			
70	160 - 170	165 - 175	170 - 180	175 - **185**	**185** + 20	205	20% or less
71	170 - 175	175 - 180	180 - 185	185 - **190**	**190** + 20	210	20% or less
72	175 - 180	180 - 185	185- 190	190 - 195			
73	175 - 180	180 - 185	185 - 190	190 - 195			
74	180 - 185	185 - 190	190 - 195	195 - 200			
75	185- 190	190 - 195	195 - 200	200 - **205**	**205** + 20	225	20% or less
76	190 - 195	195 - 200	200 - 205	205 - 210			
77	195 - 200	200 - 205	205 - 210	210 - 215			
78	200 - 205	205 - 210	210 - 215	215 - 220			
79	205 - 210	210 - 215	215 - 220	220 - 225			
8 0	210 - 215	215 - 220	220 - 225	225 - 230			

BURNING METABOLISM/HEIGHT AND WEIGHT FOR MALE AND FEMALE							
HEIGHT (in inches)	Female Age				Example Max WT with BF %		
	17 - 20	21 - 28	28 - 39	40+			
	BURNING WEIGHT				WT + Pds =	Total WT	<=25%
54	85 - 95	85 - 95	85 - 95	85 - 95	95 + 20 =	115	25% o r less
55	85 - 95	85 - 95	85 - 95	85 - 95			
56	85 - 95	85 - 95	85 - 95	85- 95			
57	85 - 95	85 - 95	90 - 100	90 - 100			
58	85 - 95	85 - 95	90 - 100	90 - 100			
59	85 - 95	85 - 95	90 - 100	95 - 110			
60	85 - 95	90 - 100	95 - 110	100 - 115			
61	90 - 100	90 - 100	95 - 110	105 - 120			
62	90 - 100	95 - 110	100 - 115	110 - 125			
63	90 - 100	95 - 110	115 - 130	115 - 130			
64	90 - 100	115 - 130	115 - 130	120 - 135	135 + 20 =	155	25% or less
65	95 - 110	115 - 130	115 - 130	120 - 135			
66	95 - 110	115 - 130	115 - 130	120 - 135			
67	115 - 130	115 - 130	120 - 135	125 - 140			
68	115 - 130	120 - 135	120 - 135	125 - 140			
69	120 - 135	125 - 140	120 - 135	125 - 140			
70	120 - 135	125 - 140	125 - 140	130 - 145			
71	125 - 140	125 - 140	125 - 140	130 - 145			
72	125 - 140	125 - 140	130 - 145	135 - 150			
73	125 - 140	130 - 145	130 - 145	135 - 150			
74	130 - 145	130 - 145	135 - 150	140 - 155			
75	130 -145	130 - 145	135 - 150	140 - 155			
76	130 - 145	135 - 150	140 - 155	145 - 160			
77	135 - 150	135 - 150	140 - 155	150 - 165			
78	135 - 150	140 - 155	145 - 160	155 - 170			
79	140 - 155	145 - 160	150 - 165	160 - 175			
80	145 - 160	150 - 165	155 - 170	165 - 180			

Your BF percentage should also reduce while losing weight. Provided is one formula for calculating your body-fat percentage. Your weight is important, but your body fat is equally important. Everyone's body mass and size is different for many reasons, and that's why body-fat composition is a very important equilibrium for the height and weight of each individual. The calculation above is based on your body equally proportion out. The chart can be used as a guideline for everyone to start.

You can reference the following websites or use your own:

http://www.wikihow.com/Calculate-Your-Body-Mass-Index- (BMI)

http://www.calculator.net/bmi-calculator.html?ctype=standard&cage=49&csex=
m&cheightfeet=5&cheightinch=10&cpound=214&cheightmeter=180&ckg=
60&printit=0&x=79&y=6

http://www.healthyforms.com/helpful-tools/body-fat-percentage.php

SELECTED WEBSITES

The following are references that can be used to corroborate my information and allow you to do further research to educate yourself on how to develop a healthy program. Remember that everybody is different. It is important to find a niche that suits and work for you and not what you read that works for someone else.

CDC, Adult Obesity, "Overweight & Obesity—Adult Obesity Causes & Consequences" (2017), http://www.cdc.gov/obesity/adult/causes.html.
http://www.free-online-calculator-use.com/military-body-fat-calculator.html
http://www.armyprt.com/apft/online-apft-and-body-fat-calculator.shtml
http://www.nhlbi.nih.gov/health/educational/lose_wt/BMI/bmicalc.htm
http://www.niddk.nih.gov/health-information/health-statistics/Pages/
overweight-obesity-statistics.aspx

These are just some of the websites that can be used as a reference to achieve your path to a healthy life. Use these websites and calculator as a guide and not the absolute. Healthy height, weight, body fat, and BMI do not show you a chart of the human body's proportions. The body's proportions are a very important part of the results. Do not let the numbers discourage you from your quest of a fit and healthy life.

PERSONAL ACHIEVEMENTS

After more than thirty years in the United States Army, I am proud to say that maintaining fitness was one of the goals I achieved. Physical training was five days a week in the army, which included an assortment of vigorous exercises. In addition, we were administered a physical fitness test every six months. The maximum score on the charts was 300. In my career, I have received ten scores between 288 and 298, six off-the-scale scores between 301 and 325, and a score of 300 for the remainder throughout my career. During my service time, I took approximately 720 physical fitness tests. These events were documented by the army.

The following are some of the achievements I accomplished outside of the mandatory physical training while in the army.

https://www.athlinks.com/event/5290/results/Event/17846/Course/26544/Bib/819

https://www.athlinks.com/event/5337/results/Event/41033/Course/60665/Bib/986

https://www.athlinks.com/event/9036/results/Event/13888/Course/20467/Bib/54557

https://www.athlinks.com/event/5290/results/Event/30044/Course/45755/Bib/246

https://www.athlinks.com/event/5337/results/Event/26345/Course/40815/Bib/955

https://www.athlinks.com/event/5290/results/Event/115331/Course/71576/Bib/340

The author's name has to be typed into these two website to see the results.

http://www.mychiptime.com/searchevent.php?id=4345
http://www.marathonguide.com/races/racedetails.cfm?MIDD=1604150322

FINAL THOUGHTS

Well, here you are at the end of the book but the beginning of your chapter. I hope that you figured out that the real formula is you. You have to love who you are and what you stand for in life in order to promote your path to a fit and healthy life. You have to ask yourself the hard questions, and remember to set your mind to accept the healthy answers.

Confidence is all you need to be successful, and if you follow the guidance I've provided in this book, all the paid advertised workouts, personal trainers, television programs, and DVDs will be obsolete in helping you achieve your goals.

Take control of your health, and be your own champion for a fit and healthy life.

ABOUT THE AUTHOR

James L. Blake Jr. is a thirty-year decorated US Army veteran (retired). He has conducted and taught physical fitness training for over thirty years while competing in ten-milers, marathons, and half marathons. He is well known for competing in races for charity and maintaining his fitness. He found that through education and training, he was able to convince thousands of Soldiers and civilians that a fit and healthy life is a great path to follow.

He also has traveled around the world to many countries, including Italy, Korea, and Germany, while observing different cultures and their ways of life and daily activities. His observations revealed that most people in Italy, Korea, and Germany are fit and healthy.

He enjoys giving motivational speeches to the younger generation to help them assimilate into society. He believes that everyone should identify and control their health and fitness.

Printed in the United States
by Bookmasters

Printed in the United States
By Bookmasters